I0757475

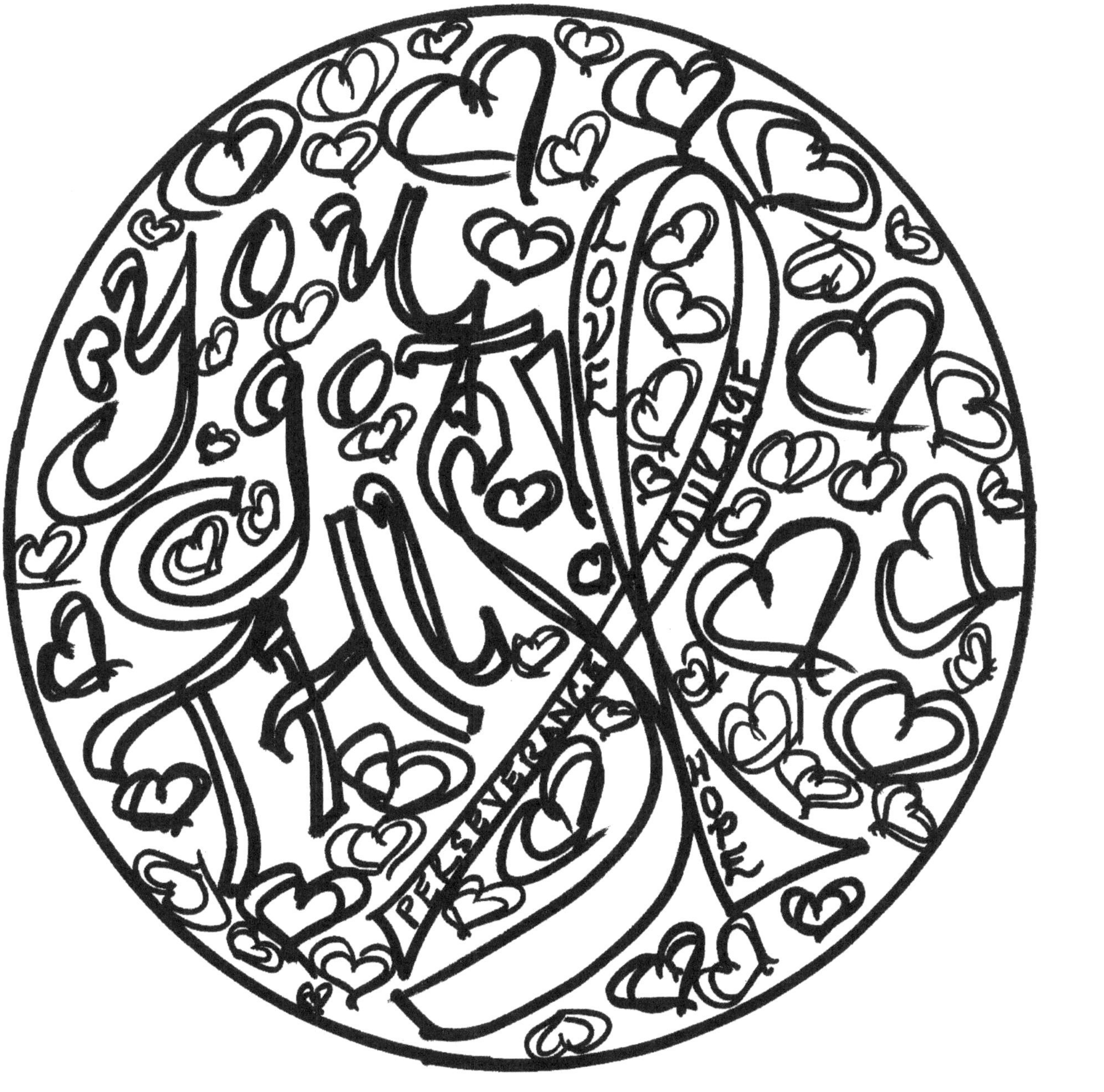

LOVE
COURAGE
PERSEVERANCE
WORK

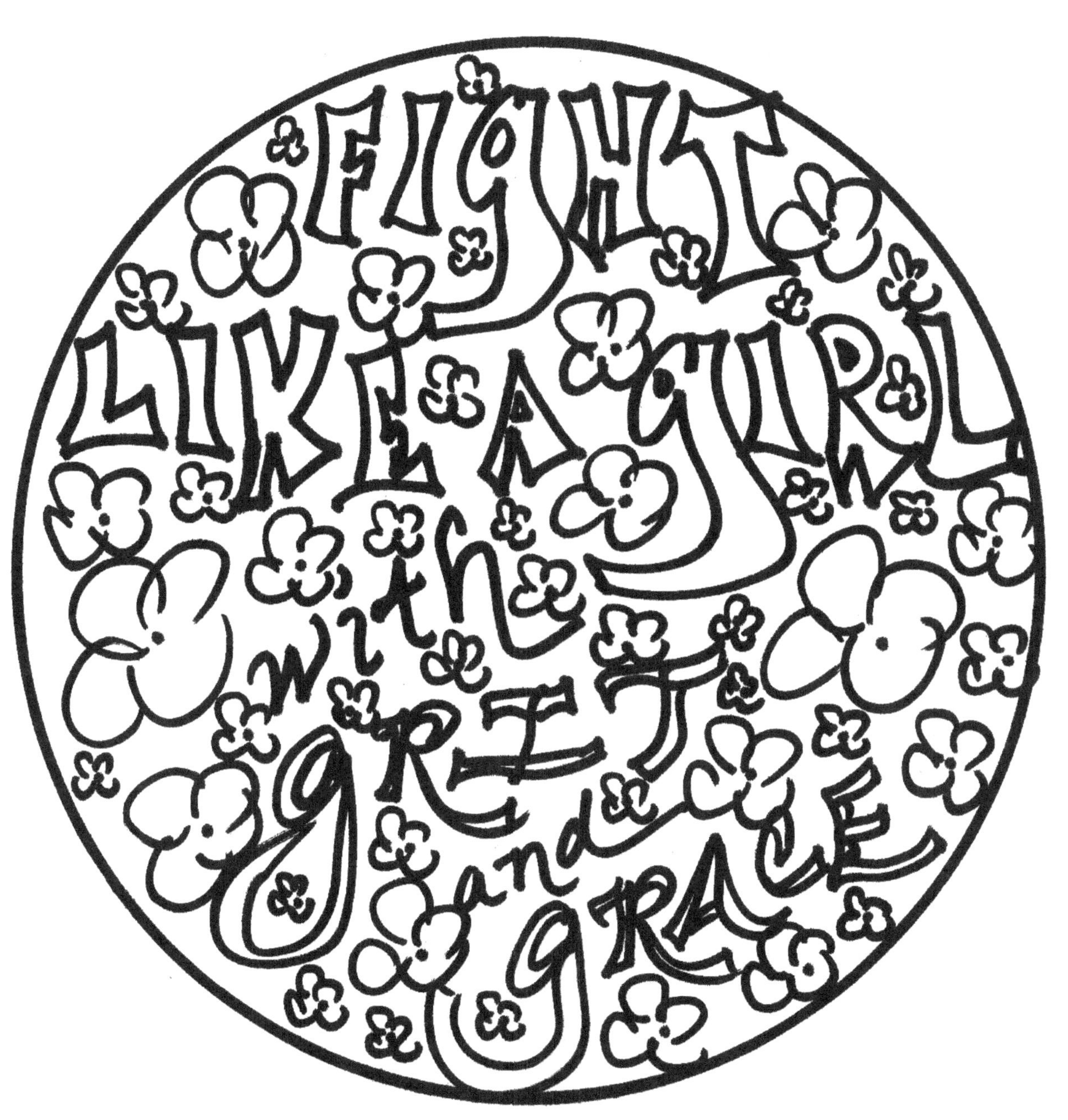

FIGHT
LIKE A GIRL
with
grit
and
GRACE

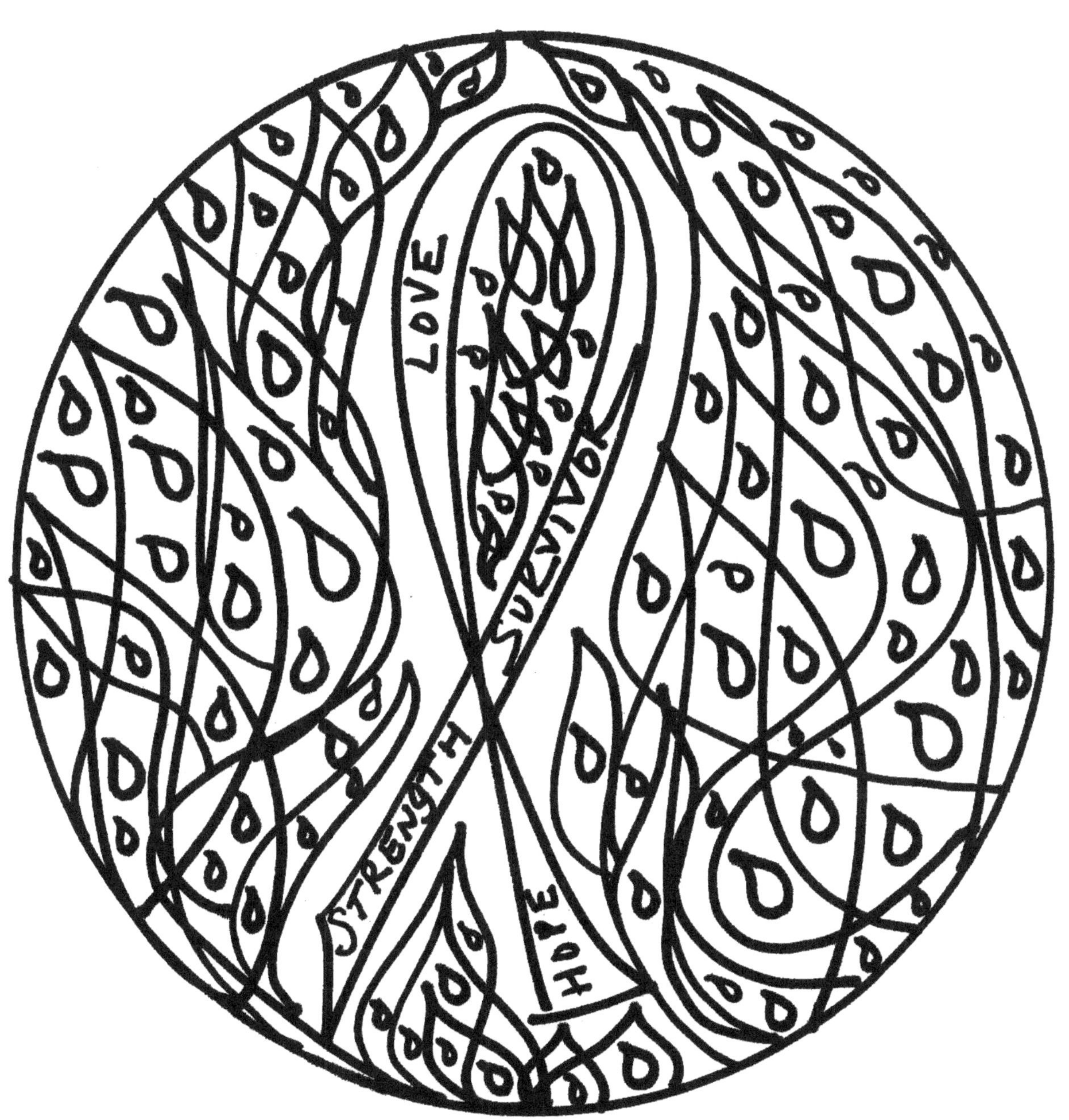

LOVE
SURVIVOR
STRENGTH
HOPE

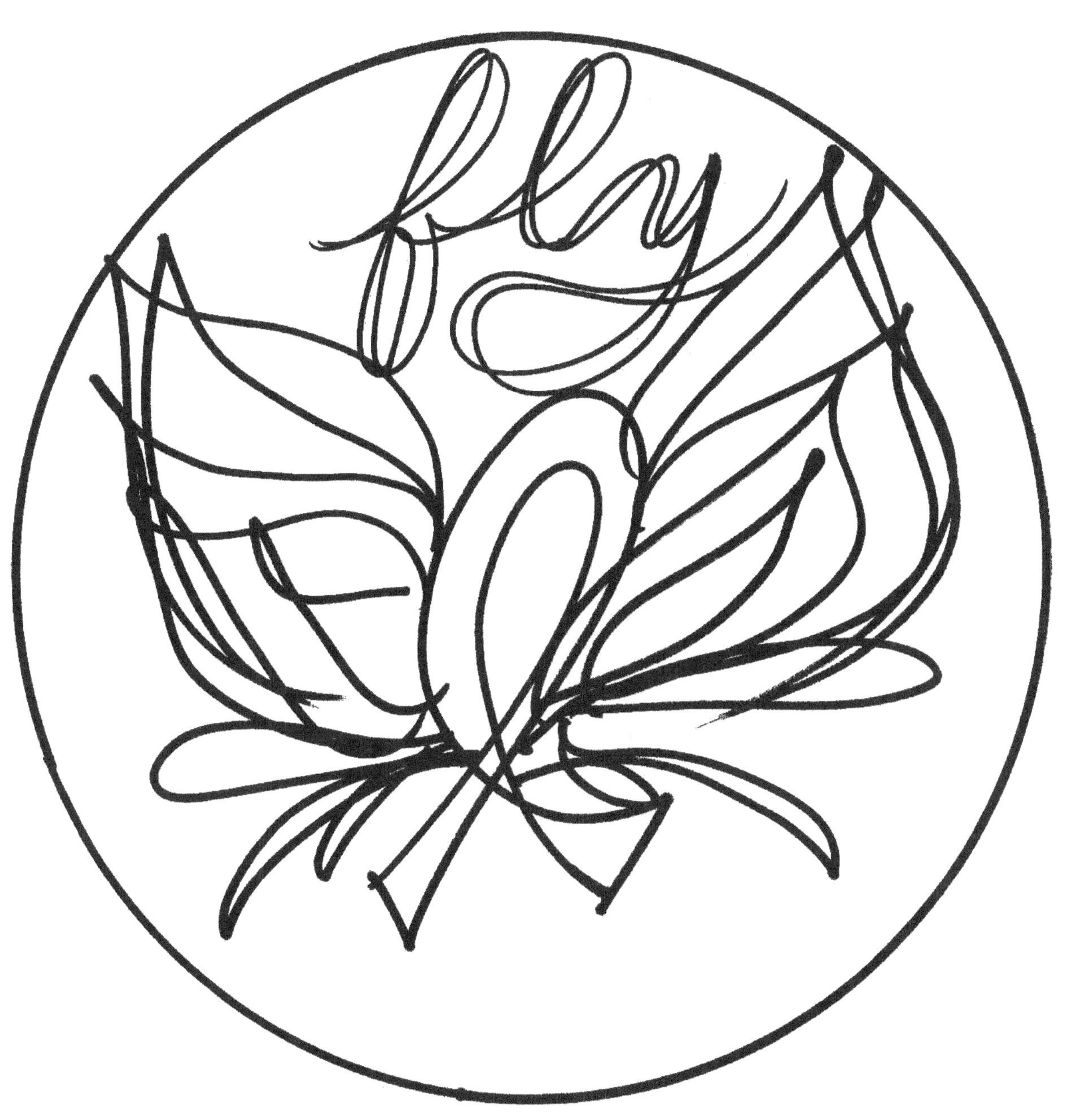
fly

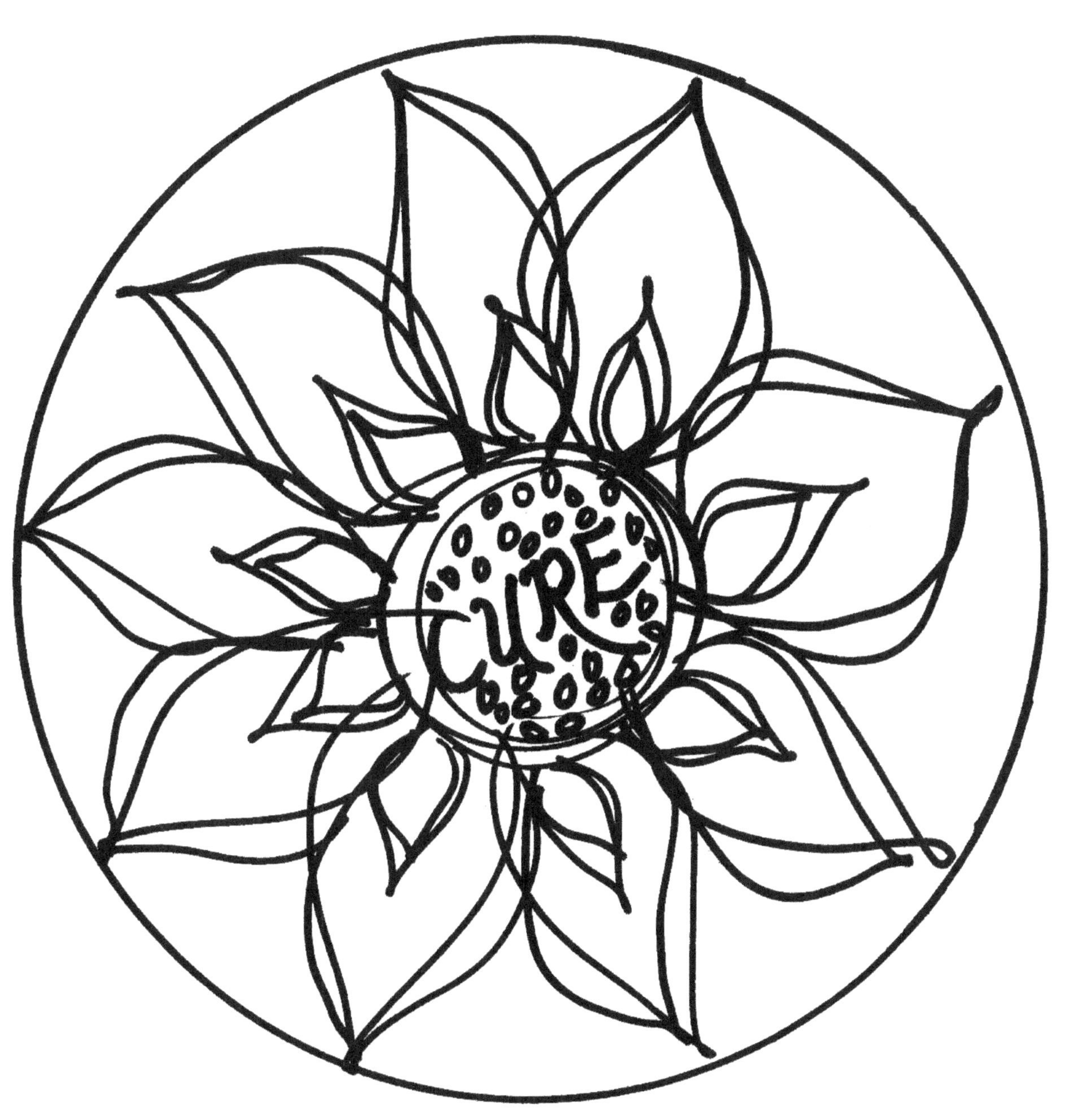

CURE

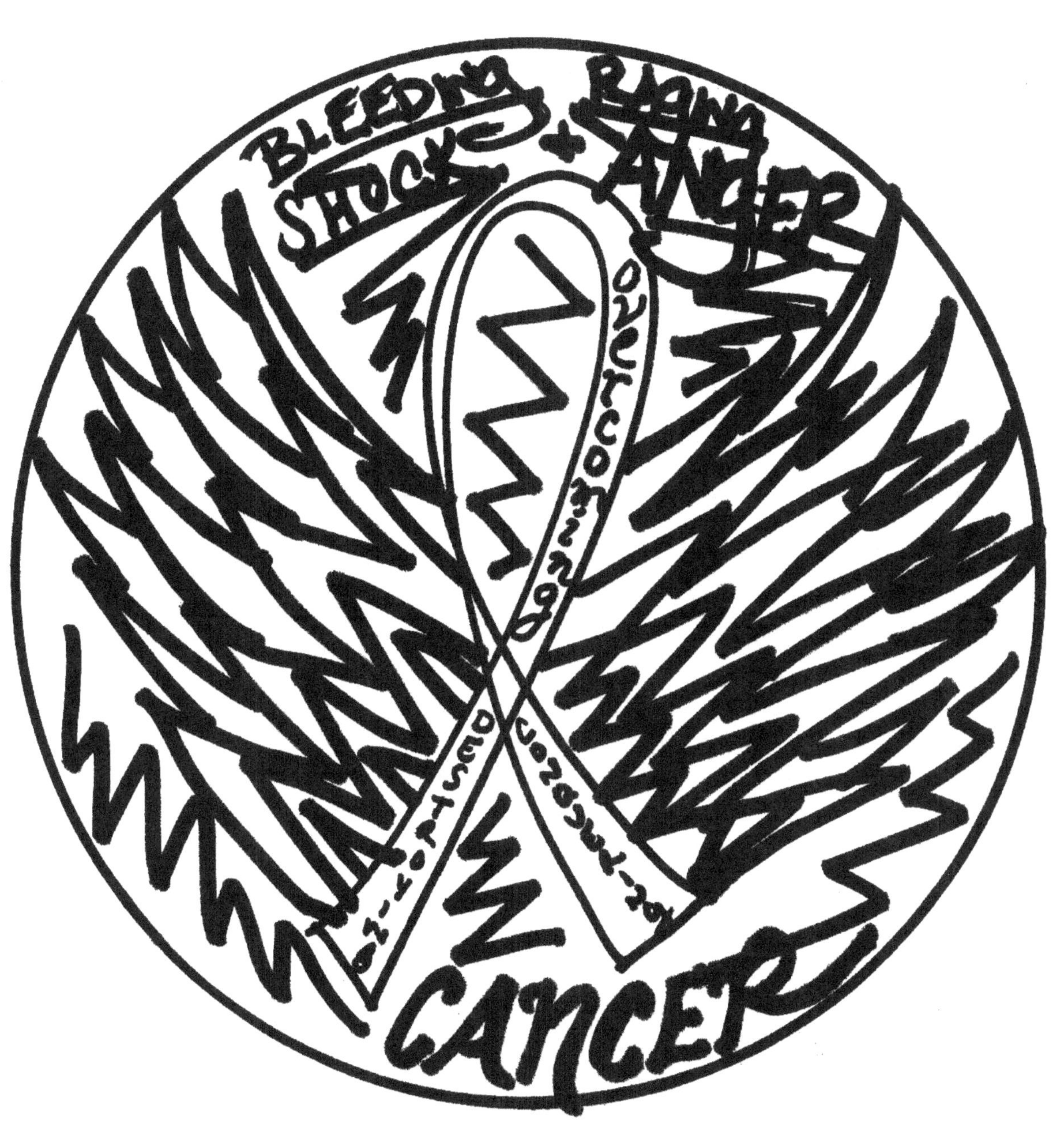

BLEEDING
SHOCK
RAGING
ANGER
OUTCOME??
OUTCOME??
CANCER

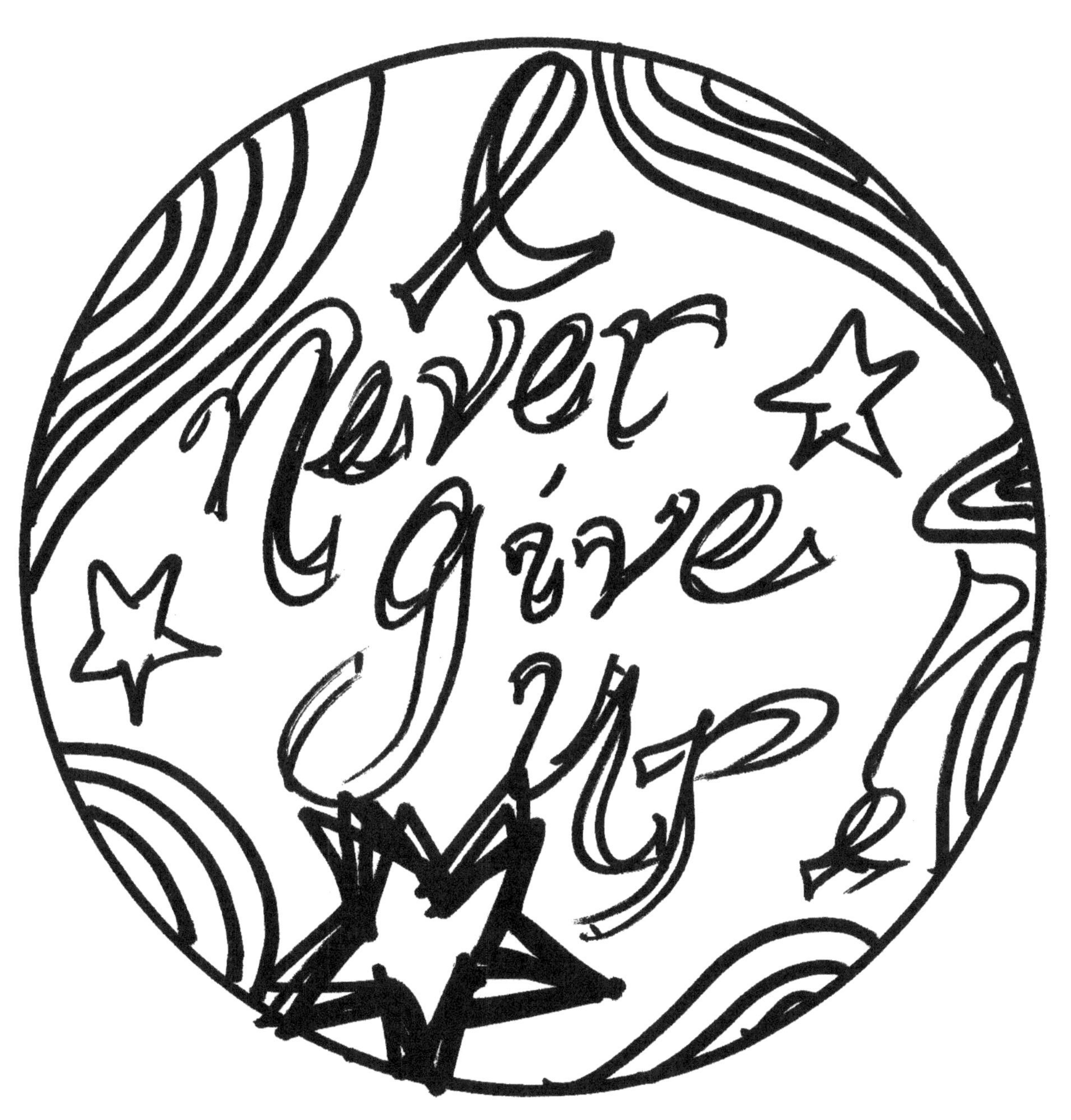
I
Never
give
up!

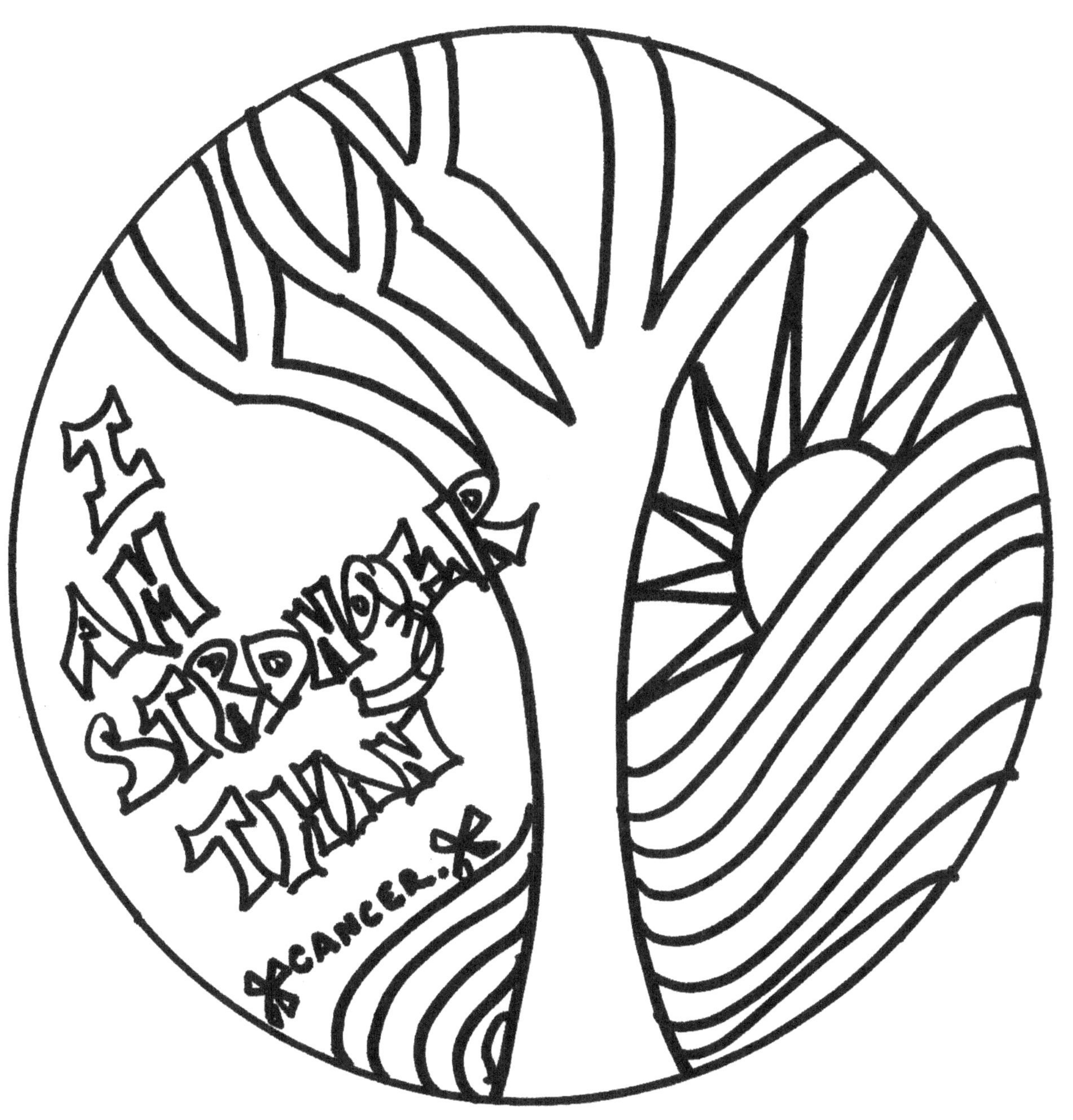

I AM
STRONGER
THAN
CANCER

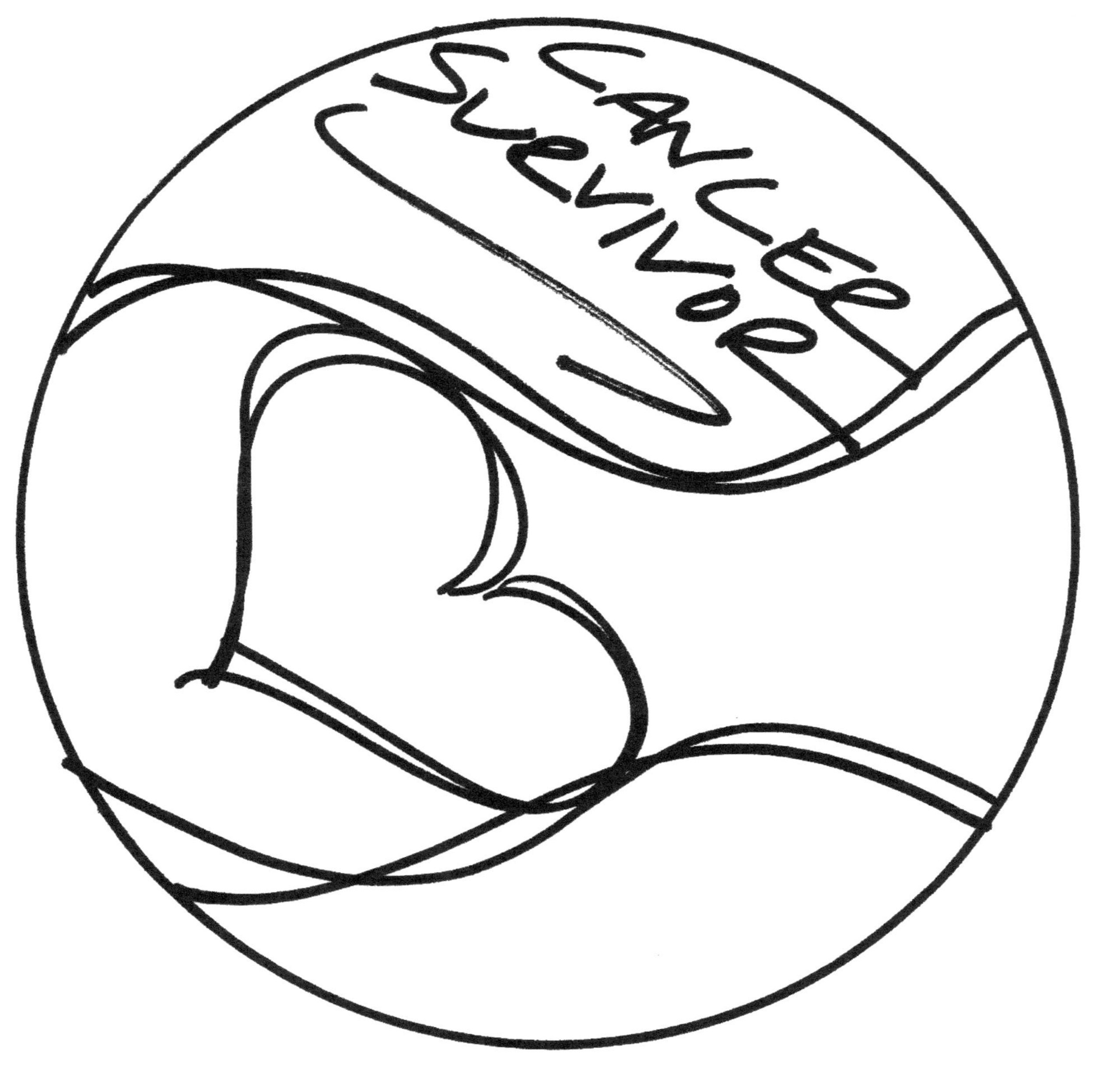
CANCER
SURVIVOR

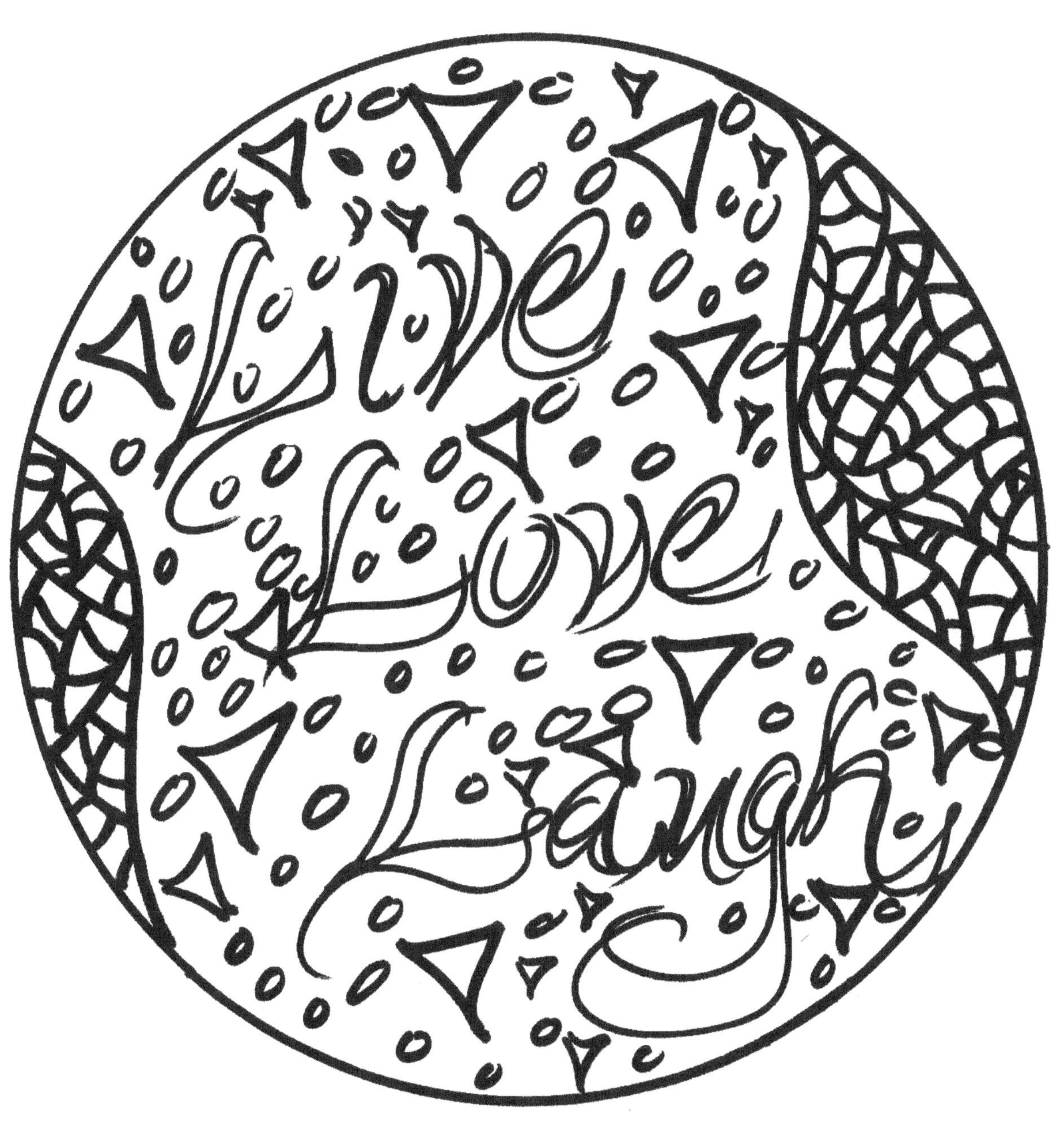

Live
Love
Laugh

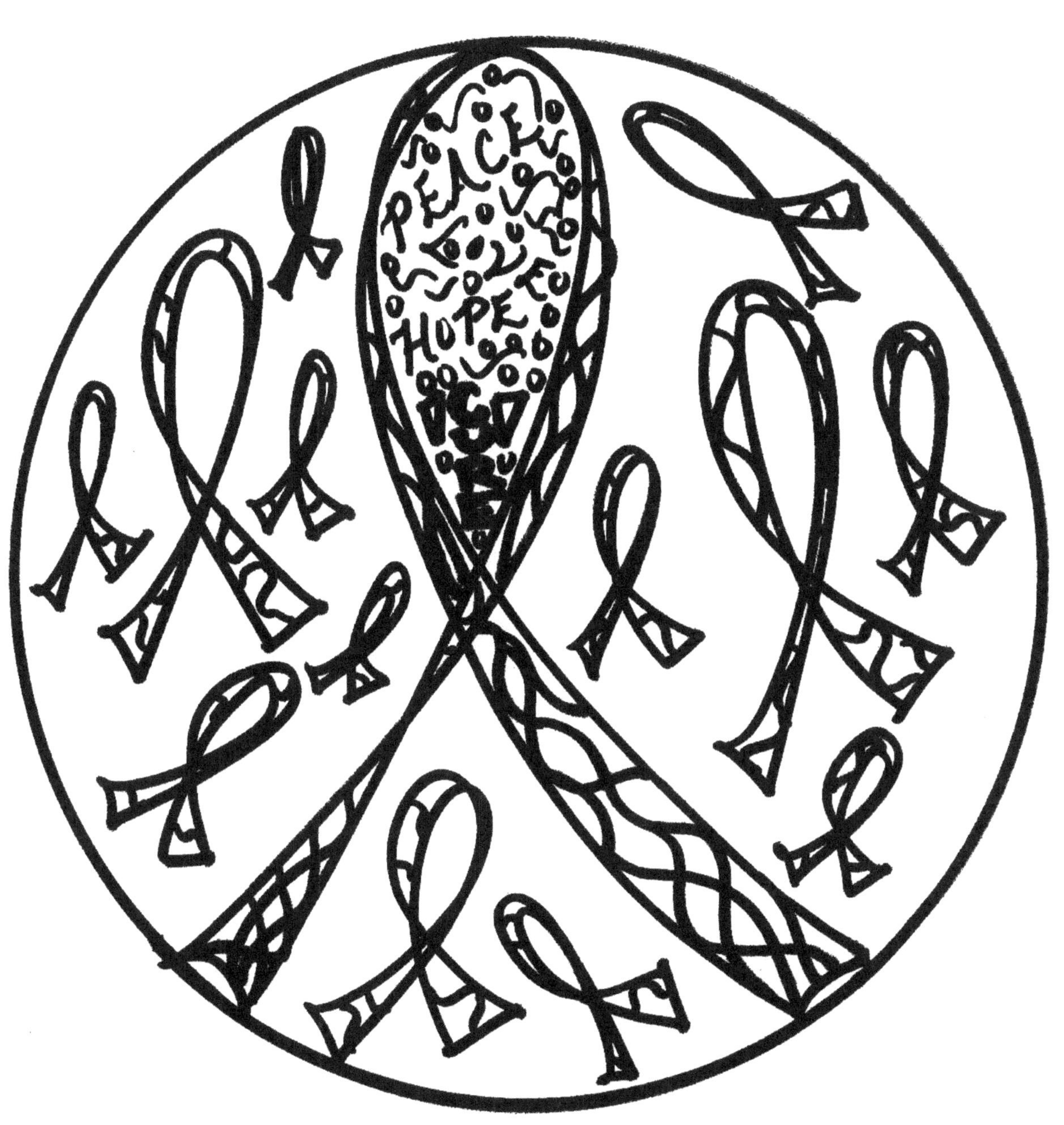
PEACE
LOVE
HOPE

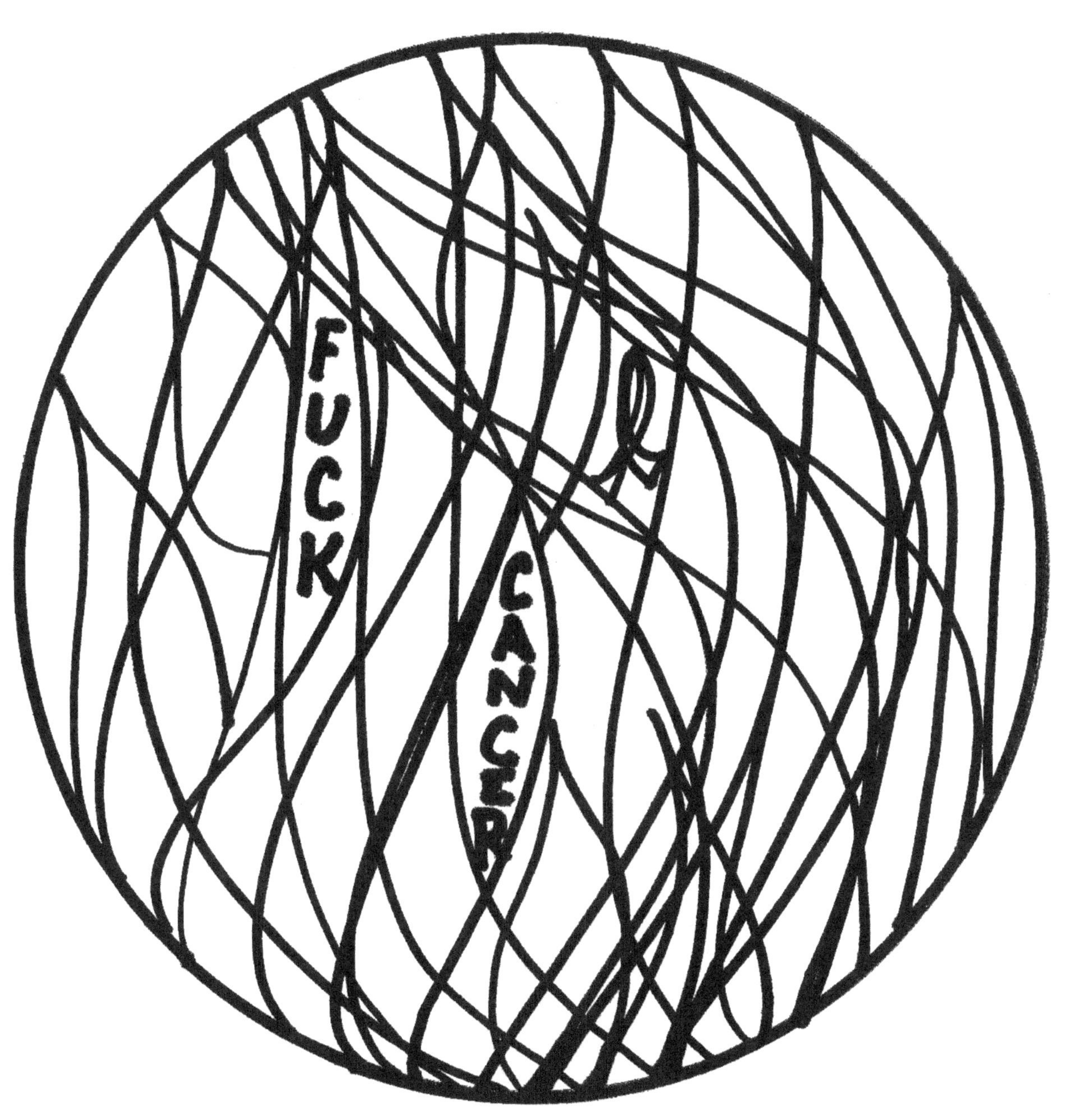

FUCK
CANCER

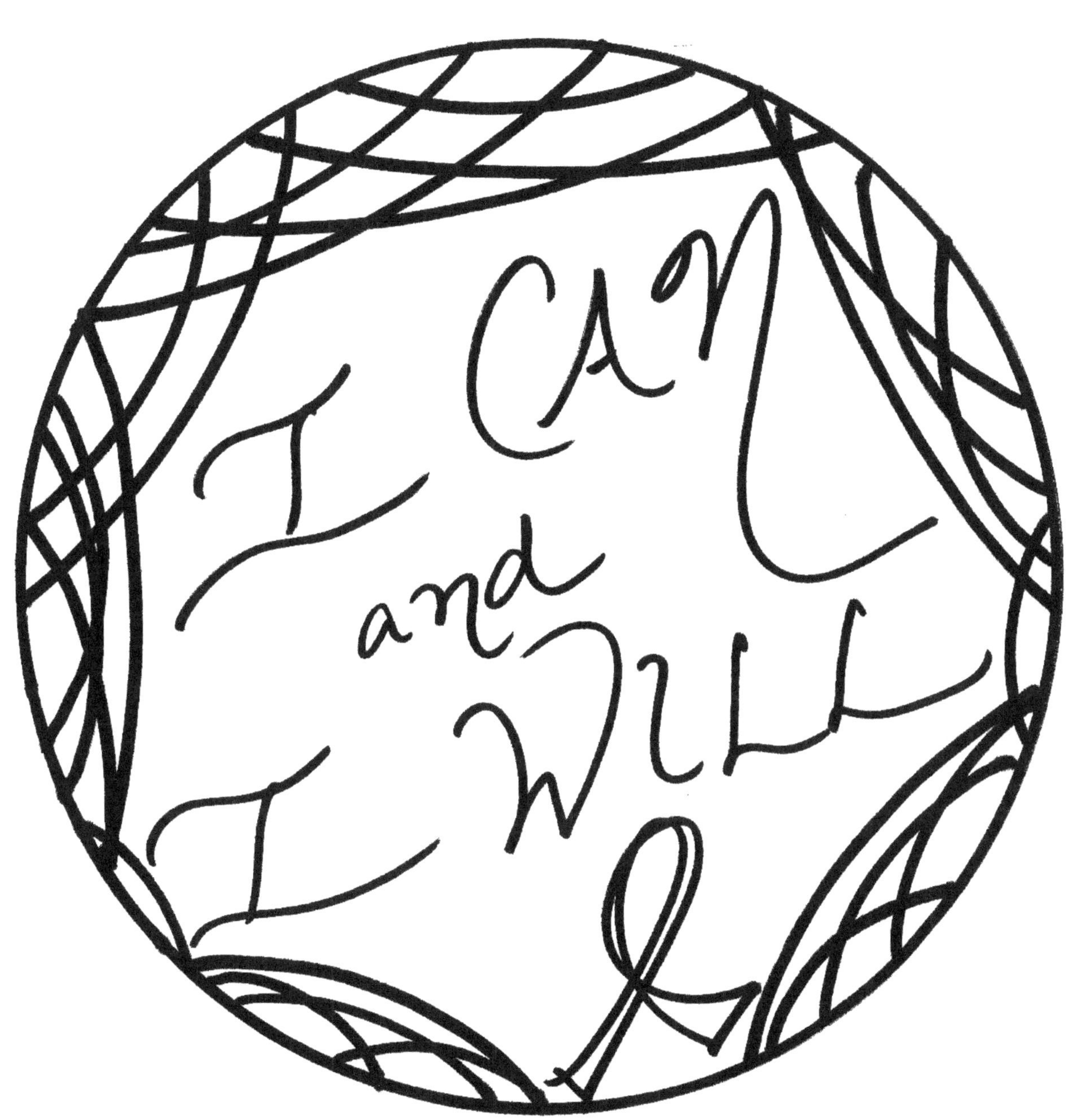

I CAN
and
I WILL

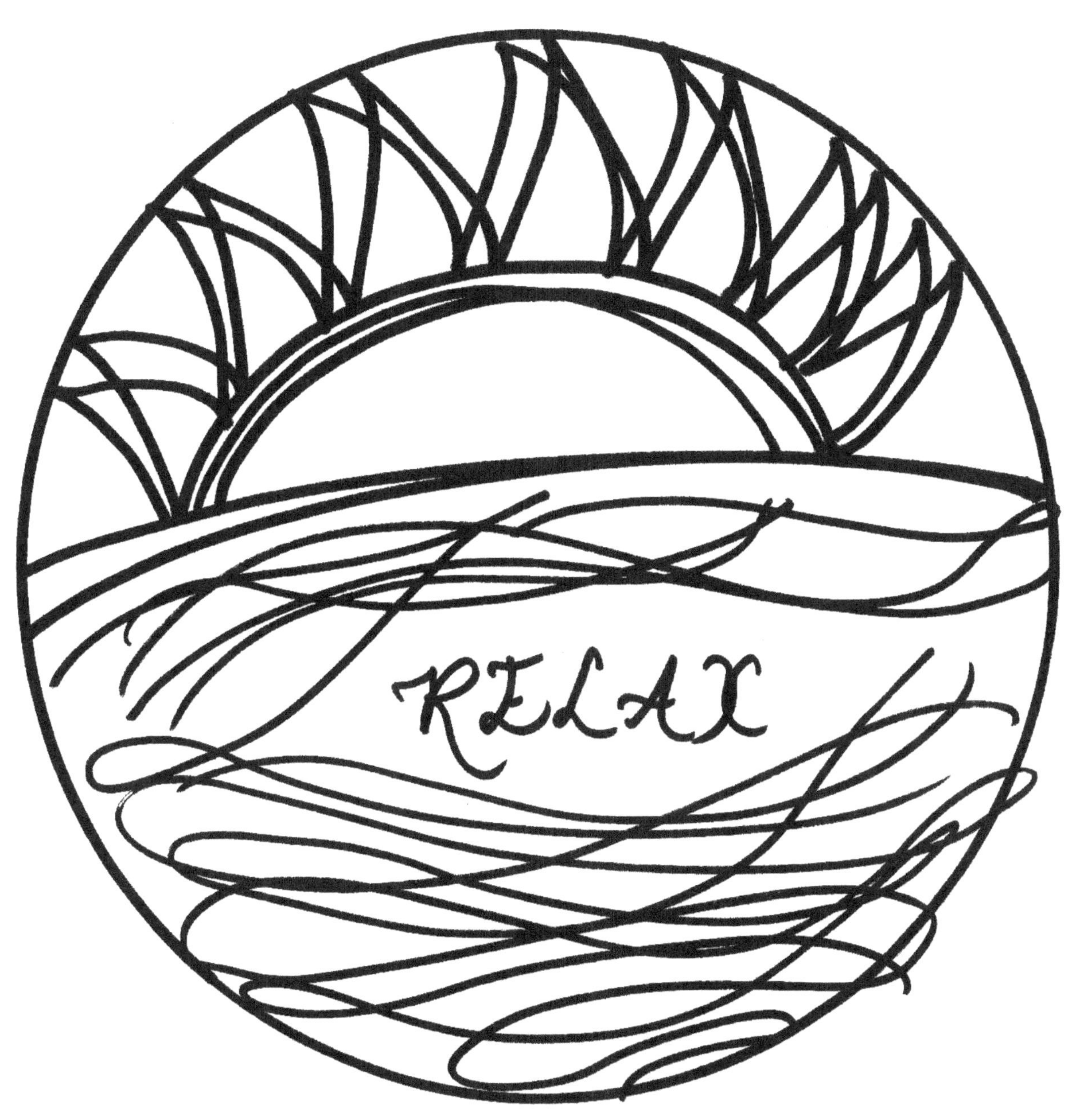
RELAX

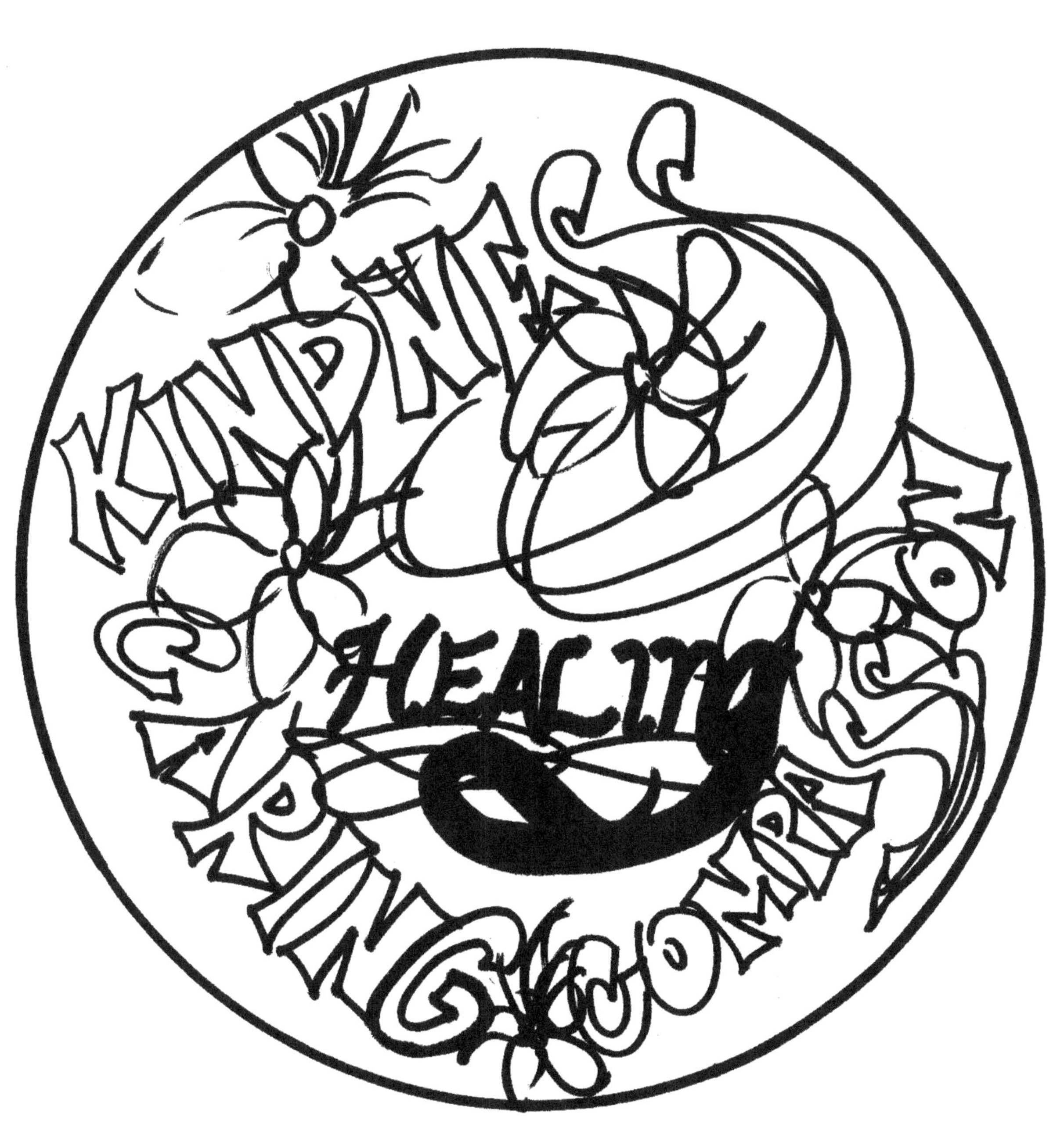

KINDNESS
HEALING
CARING
COMPASSION

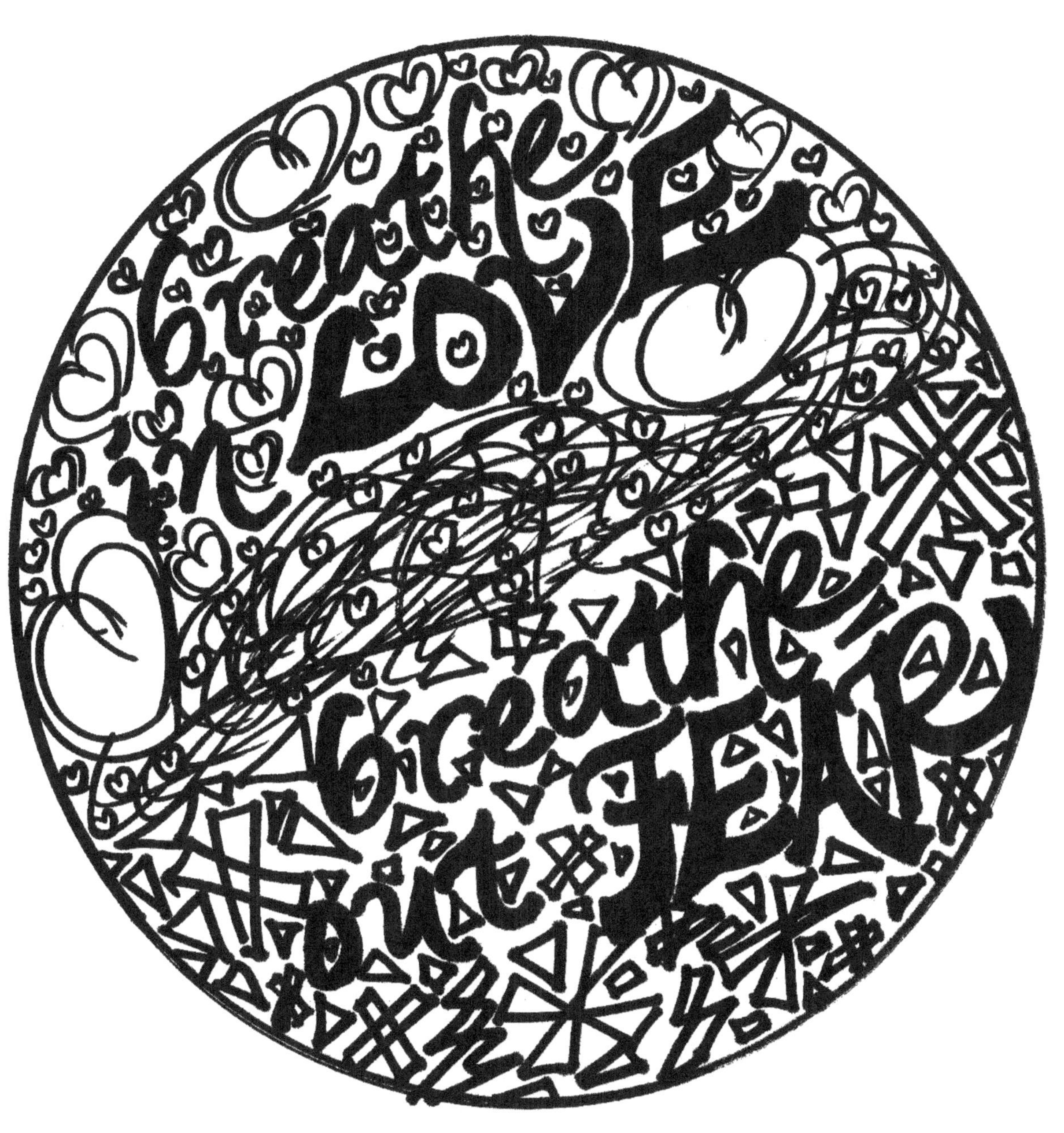

breathe
LOVE
in
breathe
out FEAR

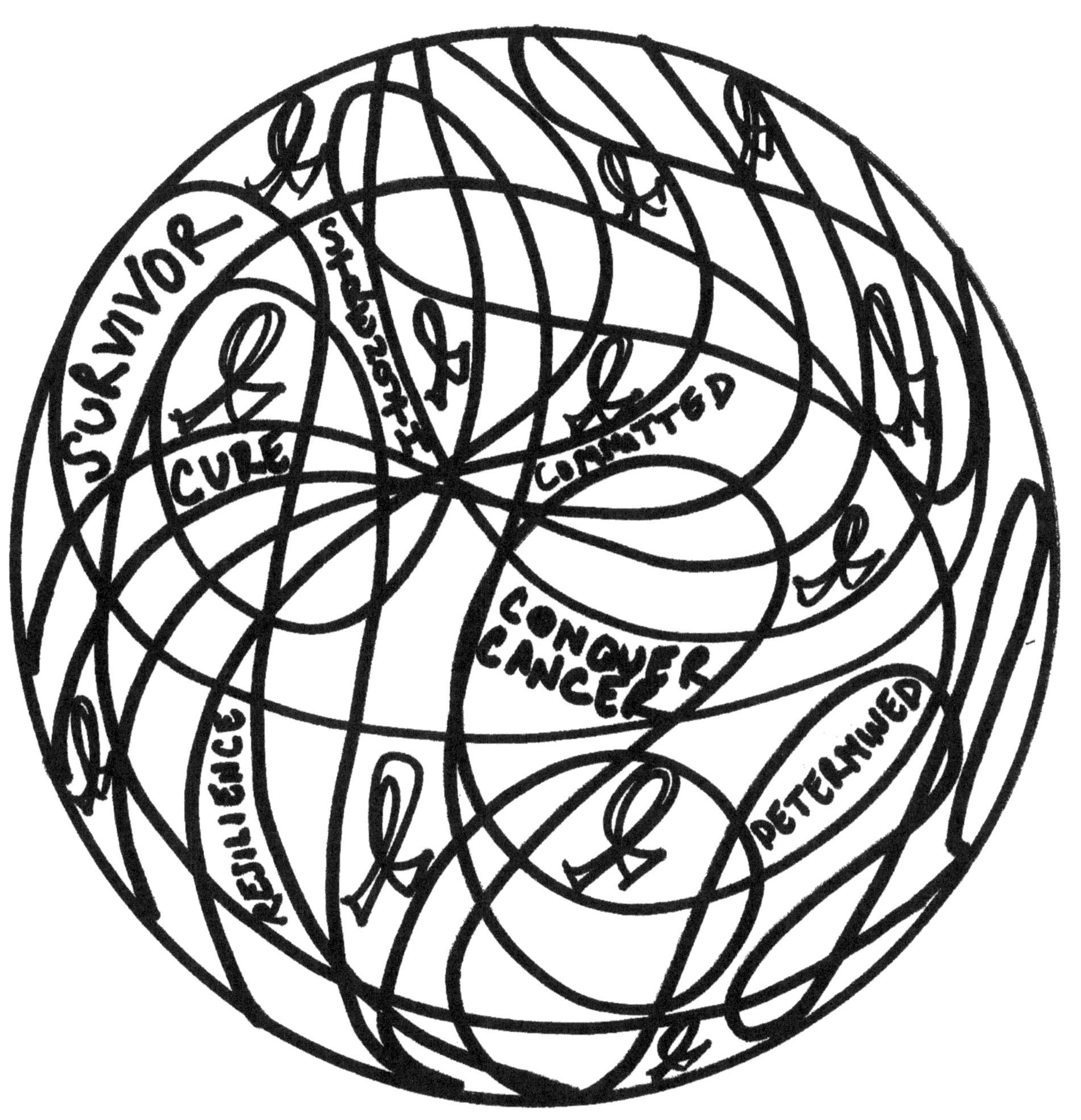

SURVIVOR
CURE
STRENGTH
COMMITTED
RESILIENCE
CONQUER CANCER
DETERMINED

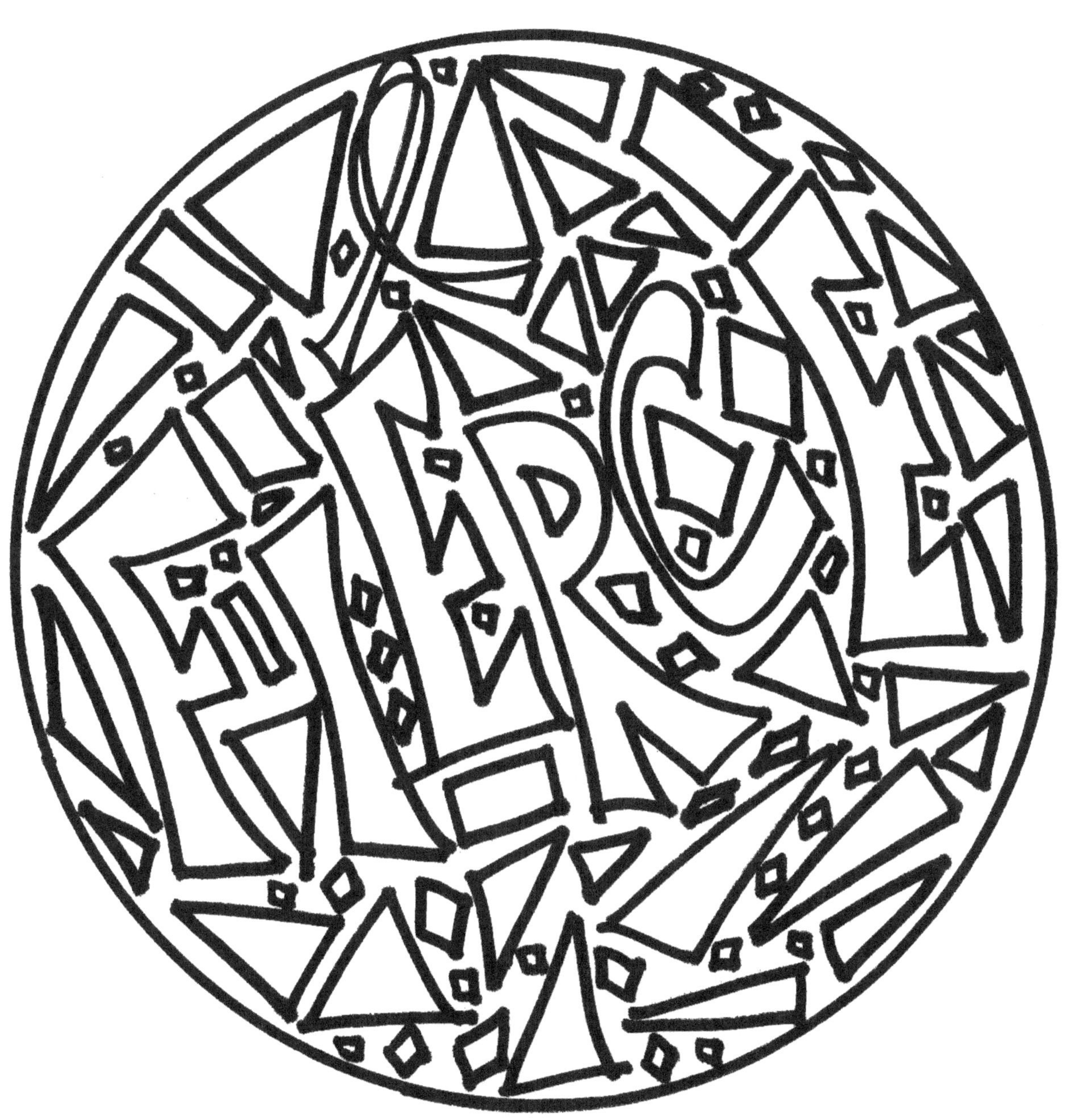

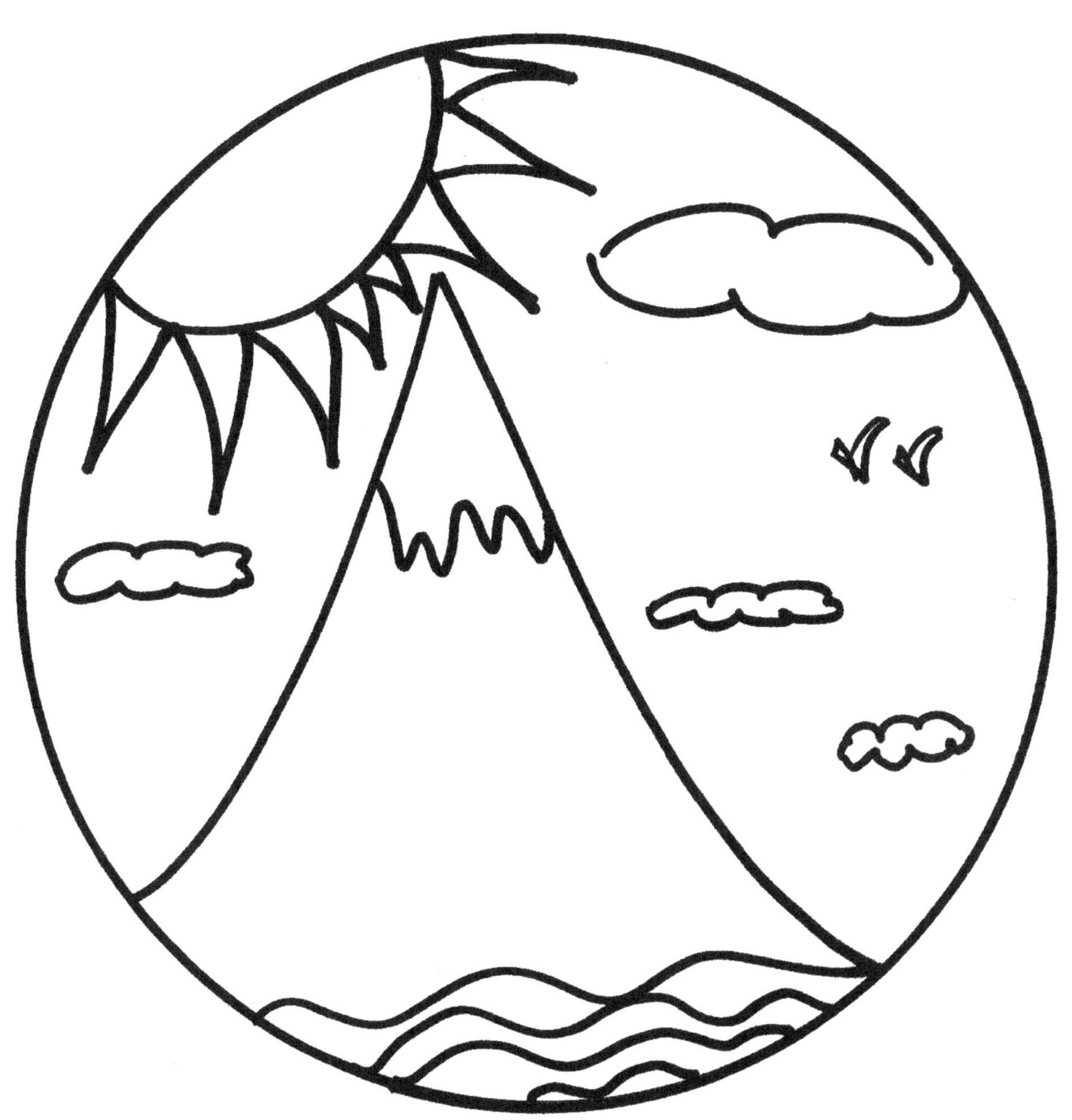

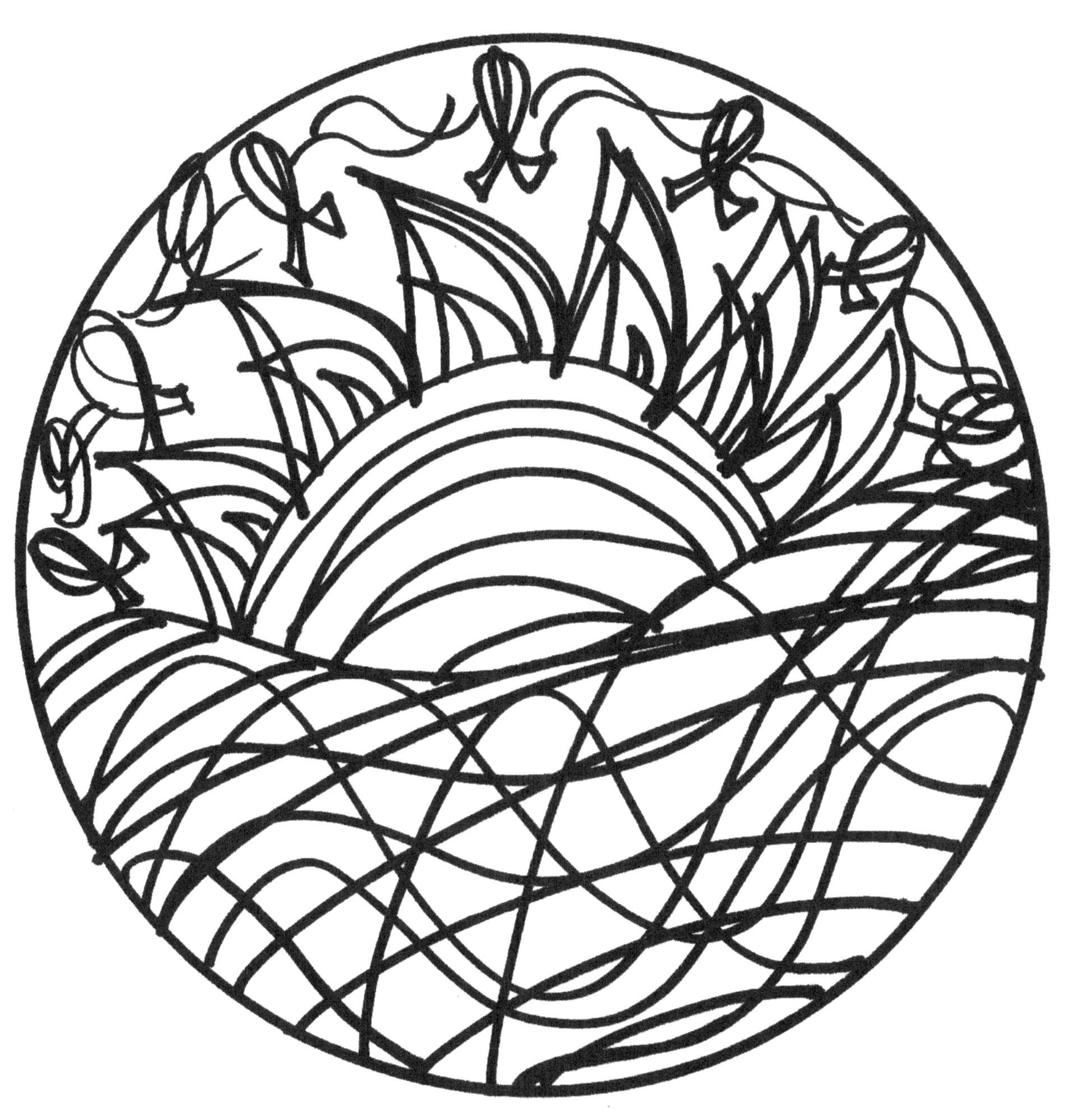

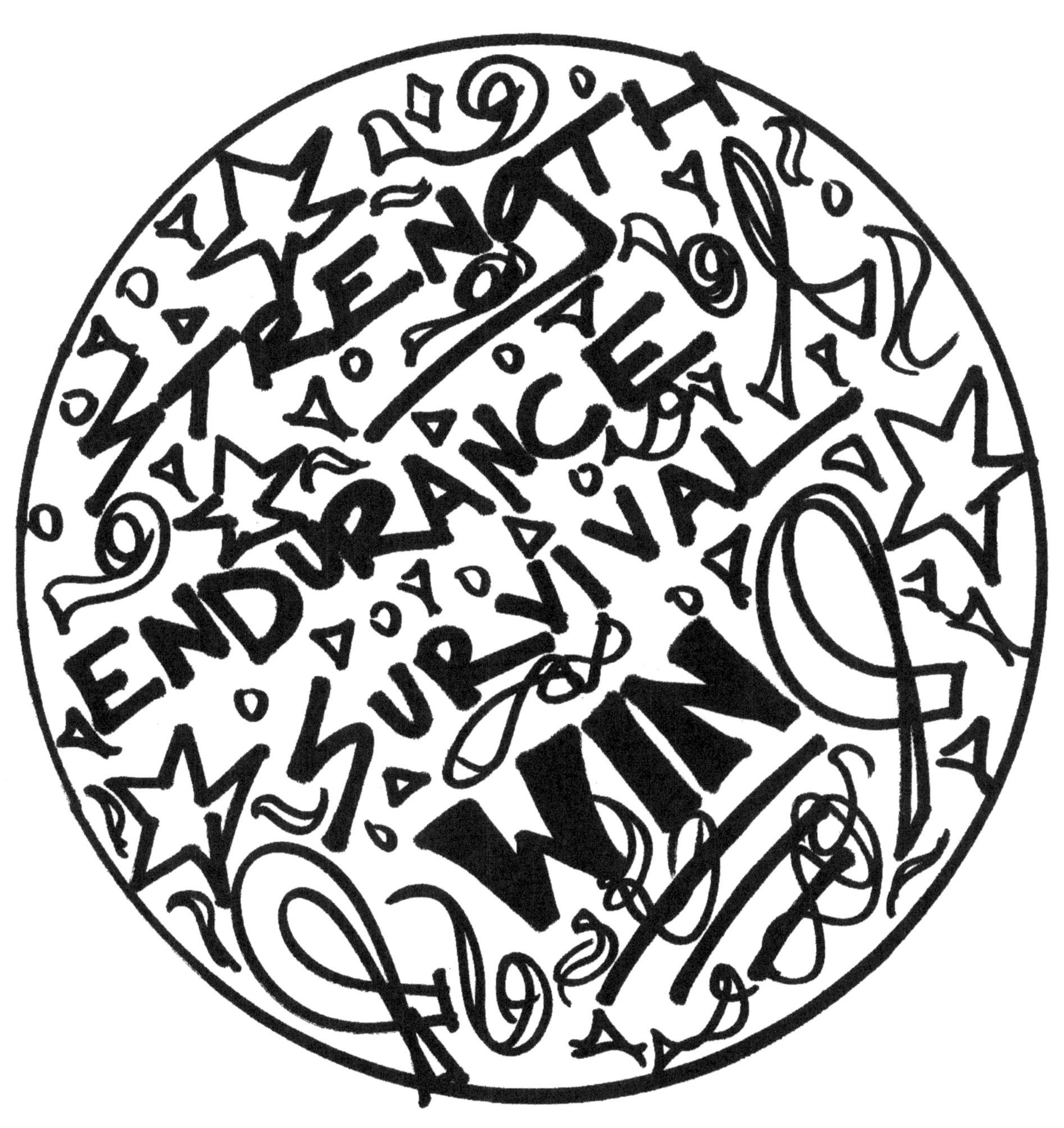

STRENGTH
ENDURANCE
PERSEVERANCE
SURVIVAL
WINNING

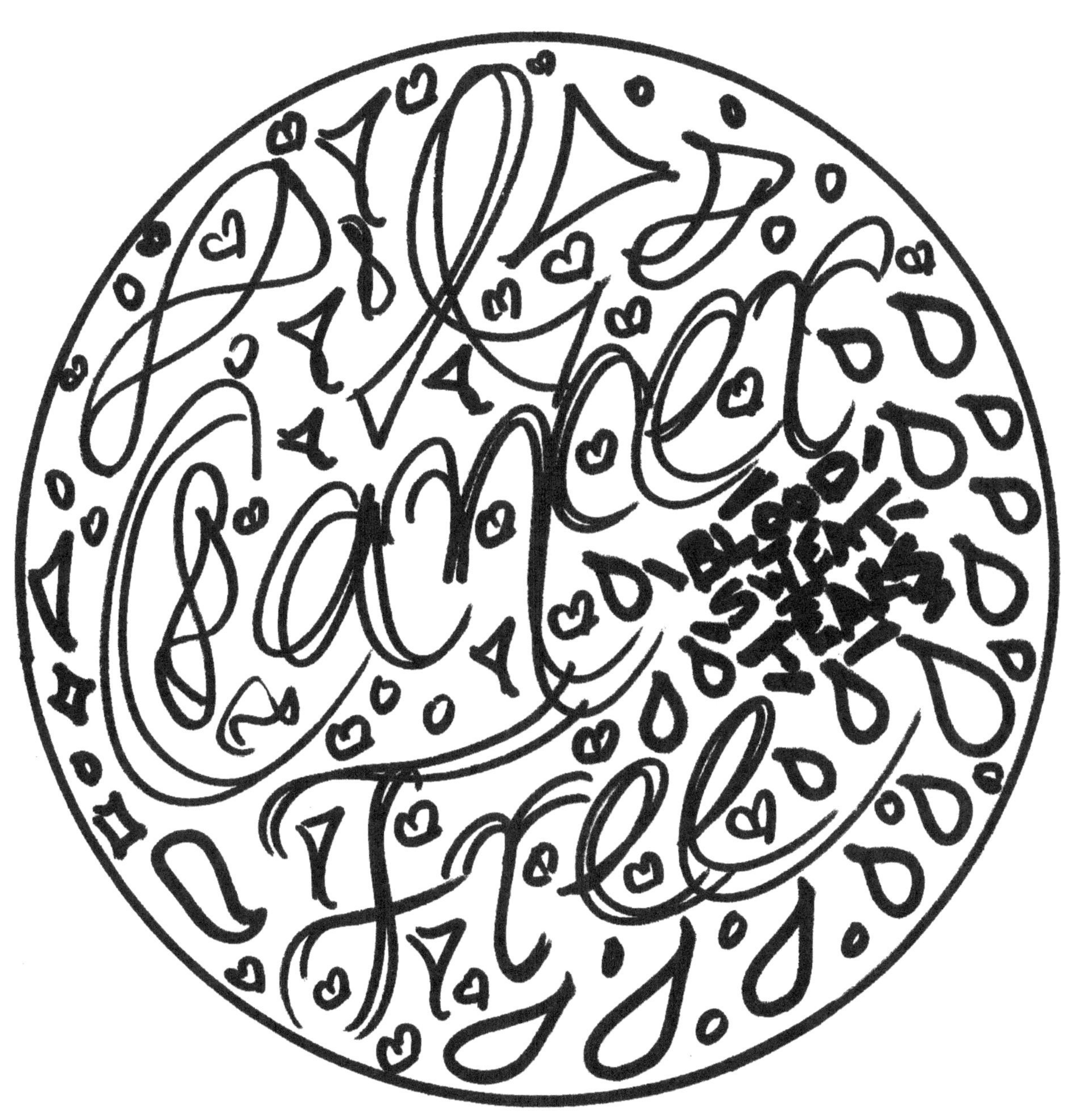
BLOOD SWEAT TEARS

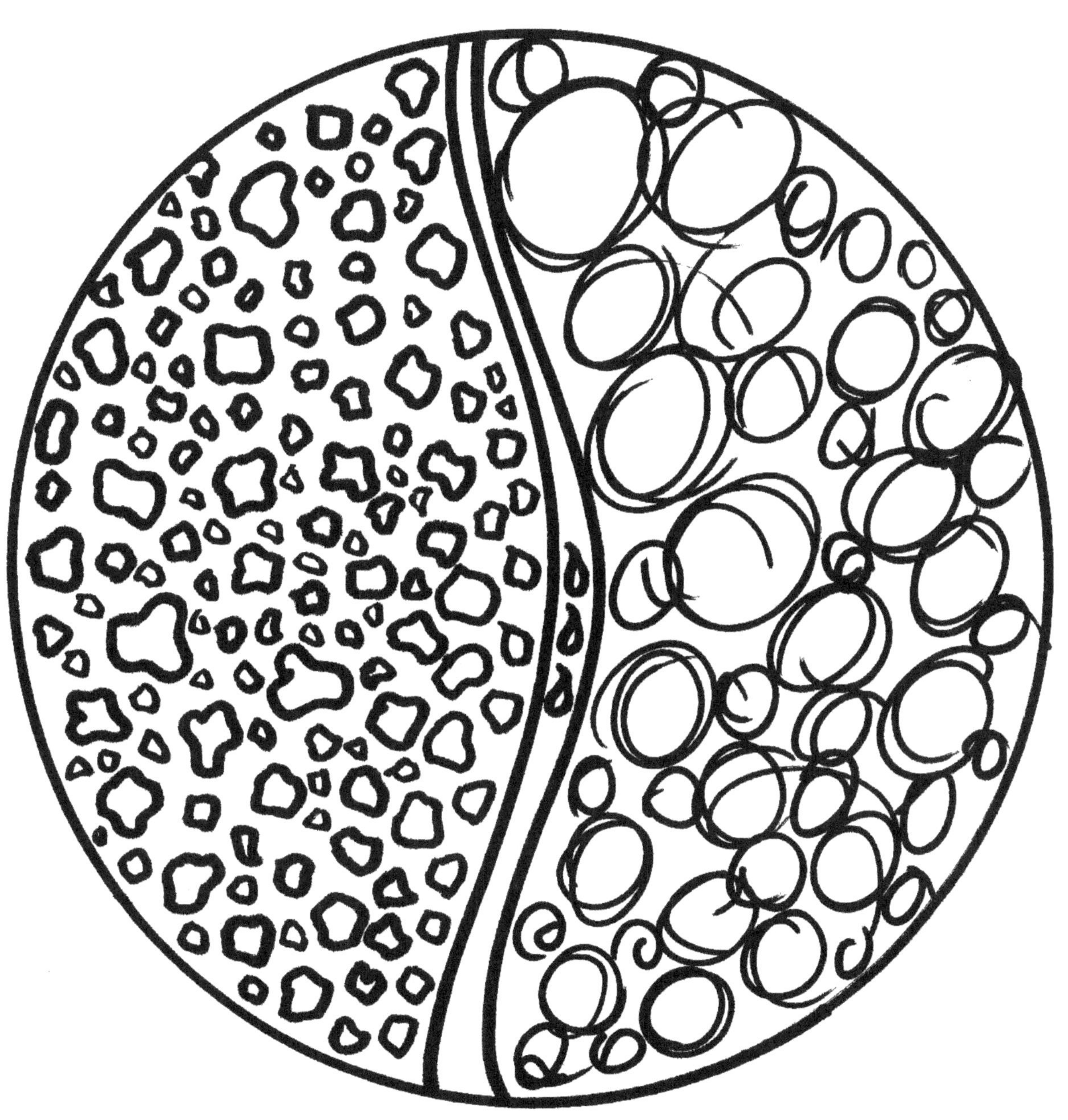

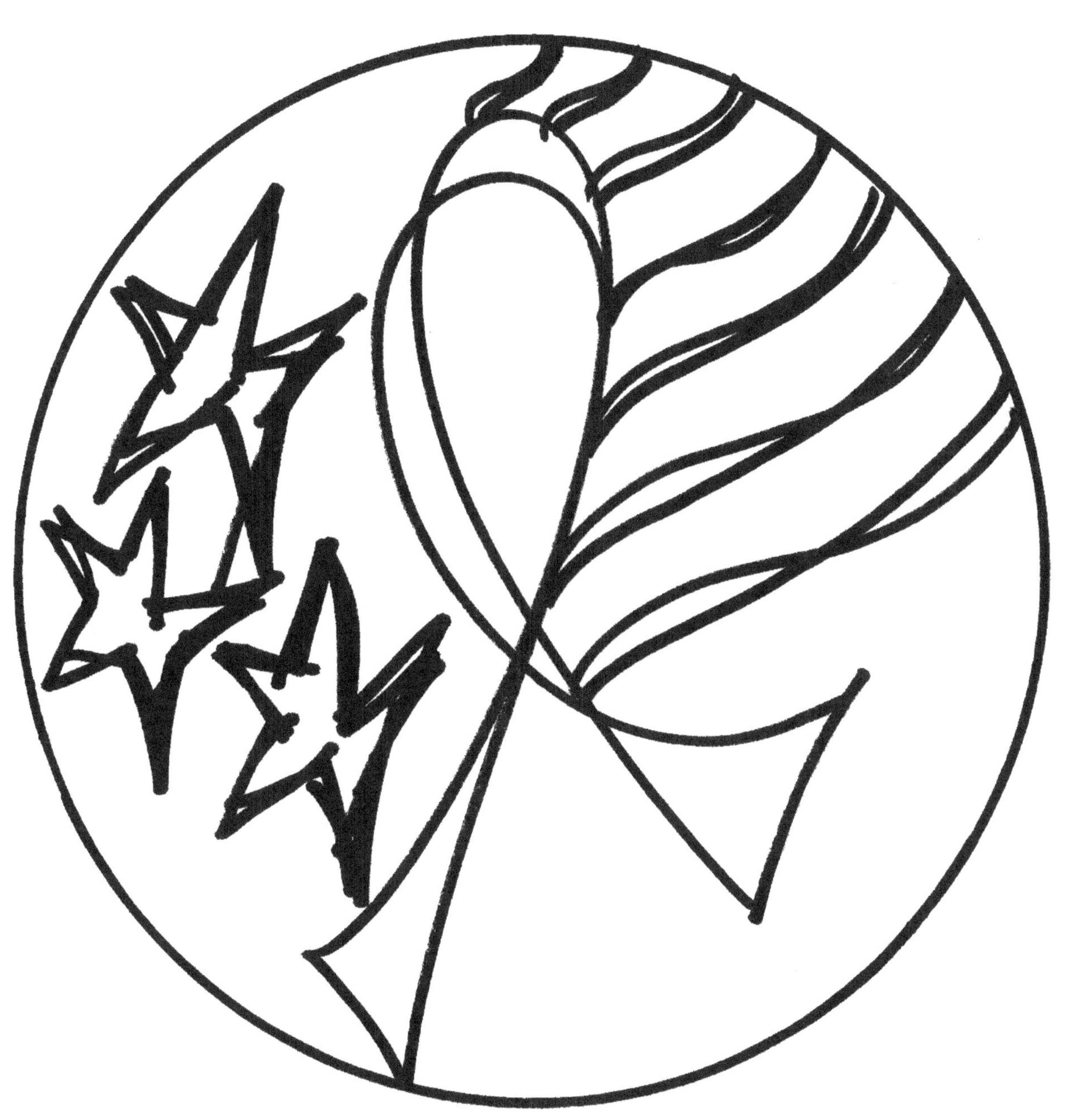

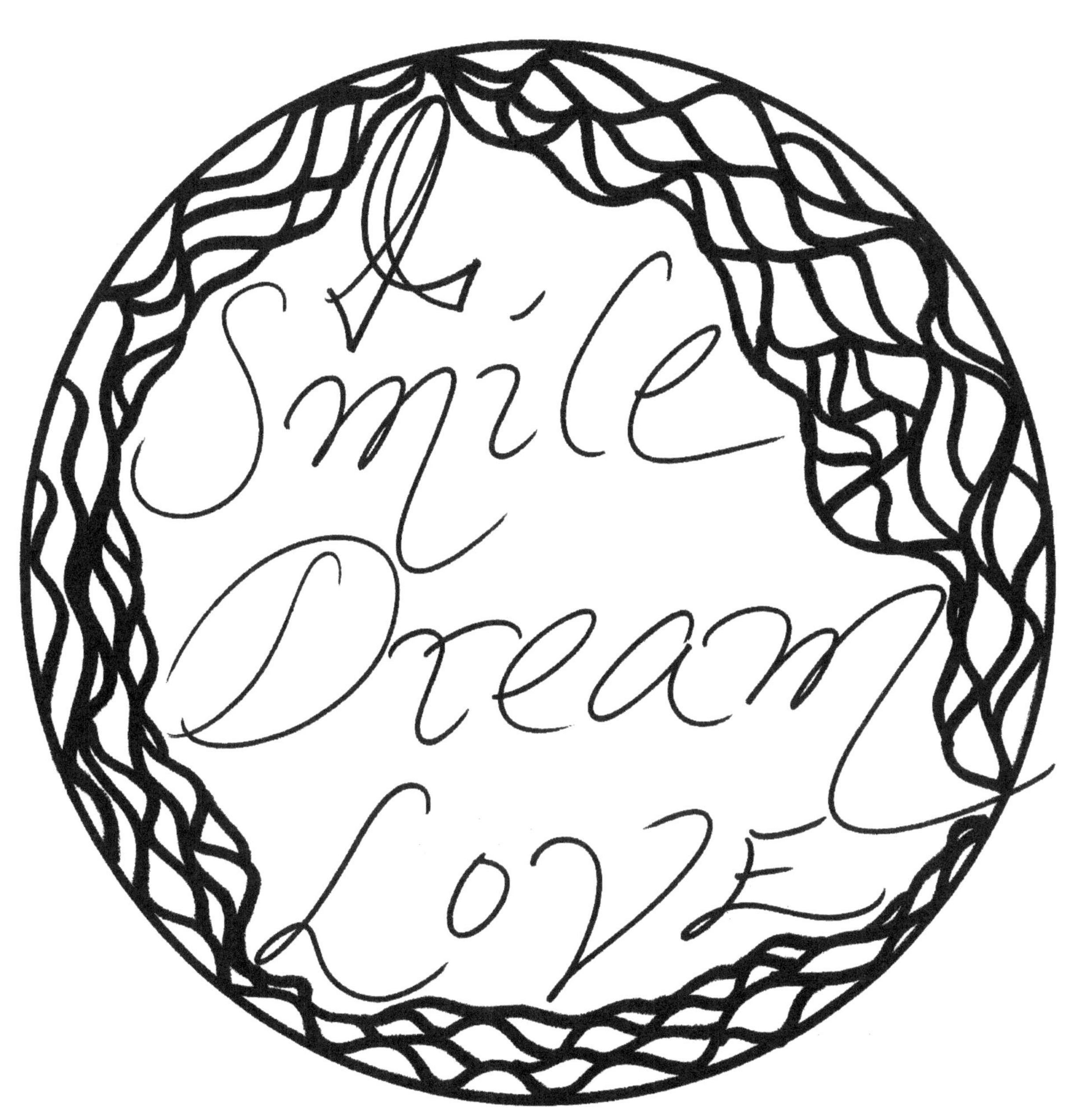

Smile
Dream
Love

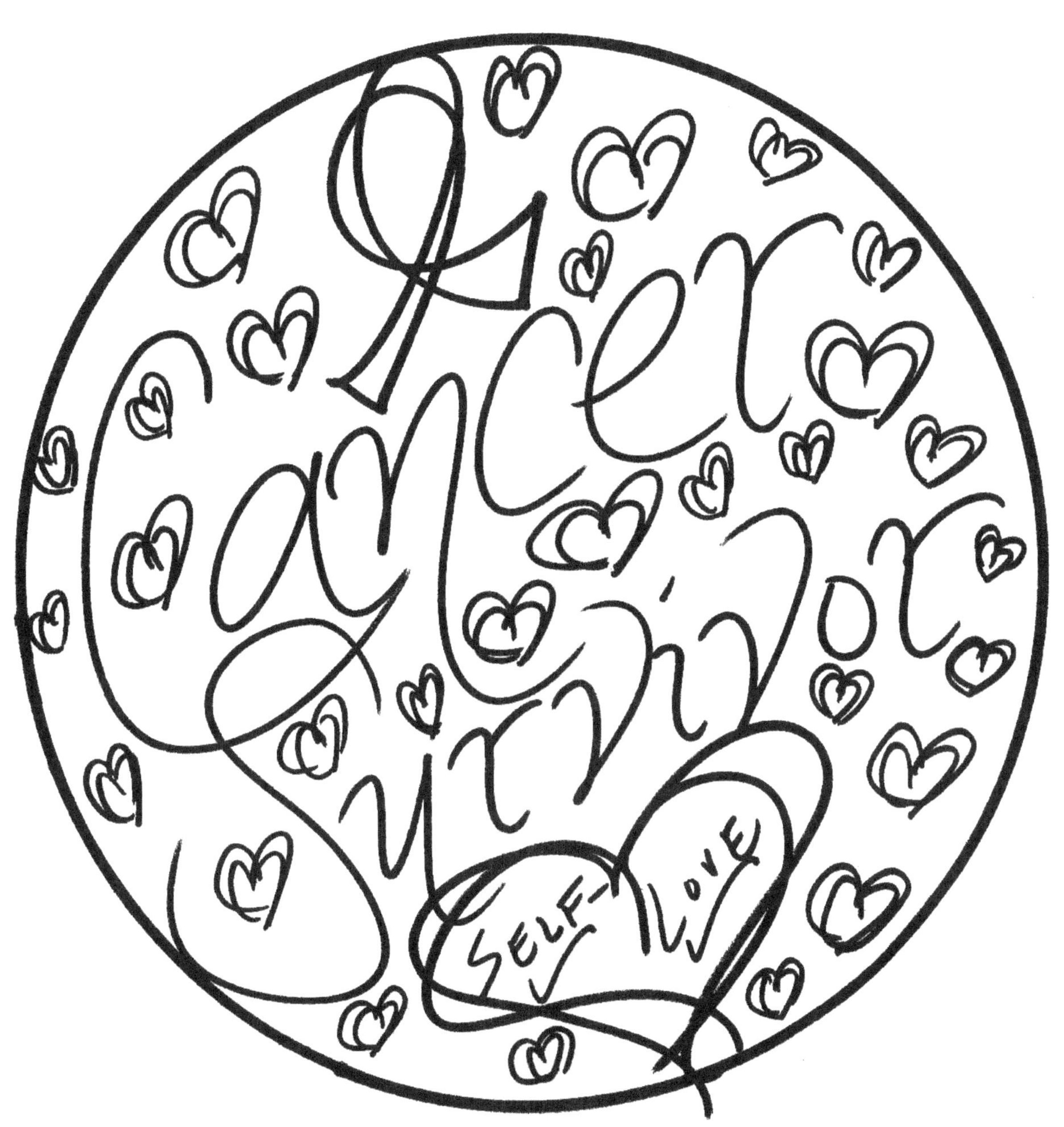
SELF-LOVE